DIABETIC SNACK & DESSERT RECIPES

Delicious Treats for kids and Adult

Shaun Renner

Copyright © 2023 by Shaun Renner

All rights reserved. No part of this publication may be reproduced, distributed, or transmitted in any form or by any means, including photocopying, recording, or other electronic or mechanical methods, without the prior written permission of the publisher, except in the case of brief quotations embodied in critical reviews and certain other noncommercial uses permitted by copyright law.

Disclaimer

The information contained in this book is for general information purposes only. The information is provided by the author and while we endeavor to keep the information up to date and correct, we make no representations or warranties of any kind, express or implied, about the completeness, accuracy, reliability, suitability, or availability concerning the book or the information, products, services, or related graphics contained in the book for any purpose. Any reliance you place on such information is therefore strictly at your own risk. In no event will we be liable for any loss or damage including without limitation, indirect or consequential loss or damage, or any loss or damage whatsoever arising from loss of data or profits arising out of, or in connection with, the use of this book.

Printed in the United States of America.

Table of Contents

Table of Contents ii

    Introduction vii

Understanding Diabetes and Nutrition vii

    What is Diabetes? vii

    Creating a Balanced Diabetes Meal Plan xi

    Smart Snacking for Stable Blood Sugar Levels xiii

Navigating Diabetic Dietary Requirements 1

    Balancing Carbohydrates for Blood Sugar Control 1

    The Role of Protein in Diabetes Management............ 3

    Managing Fats Wisely 4

    Monitoring Sodium Intake for Blood Pressure Control 5

Smart Snacking for Stable Blood Sugar Levels 7

    The Role of Snacks in Diabetes Management............ 7

    Protein-Packed Snacks for Sustained Energy............ 8

    Nuts and Seeds for Satiety 9

    Incorporating Fruits and Vegetables........................ 10

    Avoiding Processed Sugars and Refined Carbohydrates 11

    Decadent Desserts without the Guilt........................ 13

    Embracing Natural Sweeteners 13

    Incorporating Whole Grains.................................... 14

    Exploring Fruit-Based Desserts 15

    Utilizing Nut Flours and Meals 16

    Frozen Delights.. 17

Fruity Indulgences: Berry Bliss 19

    Nutritional Benefits of Berries 19

Fresh Berry Delights...20

Berry-licious Smoothies 21

Baked Berry Treats..22

Frozen Berry Delicacies 23

Nutty Delights: Irresistible Treats with Nuts 25

The Nutritional Benefits of Nuts 25

Nutty Toppings and Mix-ins 26

Nutty Energy Bites 27

Nuts in Baked Treats 28

Nutty Frozen Delicacies..29

Chocolate Lover's Paradise: Sinless Cocoa Creations 31

The Health Benefits of Dark Chocolate..............................31

Mindful Chocolate Choices 32

Guilt-Free Chocolate Treats 33

Creative Cocoa Confections 34

Frozen Chocolate Delights 35

Wholesome Baked Goods: Cakes, Muffins & More.......................37

Smart Ingredient Swaps for Baked Goods 37

Muffins and Cupcakes...41

Wholesome Cakes..45

Frozen Pleasures: Diabetic-Friendly Ice Creams 49

The Quest for Diabetic-Friendly Ice Creams 49

Creamy Dairy-Free Delights 50

Almond Chocolate Chip Ice Cream: 51

Classic Favorites, Redefined.......................................52

Strawberry Banana Nice Cream:......................................53

Mint Chocolate Avocado Ice Cream: 54

Chapter 10:..56

No-Bake Delicacies: Quick and Easy Desserts..........................56

The Joys of No-Bake Desserts 56

Peanut Butter Oat Energy Balls...57

Almond Date Energy Balls..58

Delightful Chilled Puddings 59

Chia Seed Pudding: 60

Avocado Chocolate Pudding 61

Refreshing Fruit Parfaits...62

Mixed Berry Yogurt Parfait 62

Tropical Fruit Coconut Parfait 63

Chapter 11:..65

Kid-Friendly Snacks: Fun and Healthy Bites 65

The Importance of Kid-Friendly Snacks 65

Keeping Energy Levels Stable..65

Supporting Growth and Development: 66

Wholesome Fruit Treats..66

Apple Sandwiches 67

Creative Veggie Delights 68

Veggie "Sushi" Rolls 68

Veggie Rainbow Sticks...69

Protein-Packed Nibbles..70

Cheese and Turkey Roll-Ups 70

Chickpea Snack Mix:...71

Comforting Classics: Diabetic Desserts with a Twist.....................73

Redefining All-Time Favorites 73

Apple Crisp with Oat Topping: 73

Crustless Pumpkin Pie 75

Guilt-Free Chocolate Treats 76

Chocolate Avocado Pudding 76

Chocolate Chia Seed Pudding: 78

Healthier Twists on Childhood Favorites 79

Banana-Oat Cookies: 79

Yogurt Berry Parfaits: 81

International Flavors: Global Diabetic Dessert Recipes 83

Embracing the Richness of Asian Desserts 83

Mango Sticky Rice Pudding: 83

Fresh ripe mango slices for topping 84

Matcha Green Tea Mochi: 85

Celebrating the Flavors of the Mediterranean 86

Greek Yogurt with Honey and Pistachios: 87

Orange and Almond Cake (Gluten-Free) 87

Exploring the Spice of Indian Sweets 89

Coconut Ladoo: 89

Chia Kheer (Indian Rice Pudding with a Twist): 90

Energizing Snacks: Sustaining Your Day with Goodness 92

The Importance of Energizing Snacks 92

Balancing Blood Sugar Levels: 92

Combating Midday Slumps: 93

Wholesome Fruit and Nut Combos 93

Apple Slices with Almond Butter: 93

Banana with Peanut Butter and Chia Seeds 94

Protein-Packed Snack Ideas 94

Hard-Boiled Eggs with Baby Carrots 94

Greek Yogurt with Berries and Nuts 95

Wholesome Snacks on the Go 95

Quick and Tasty Snack Recipes 97

Avocado and Tomato Toast: 98

Veggie Hummus Wrap 98

Celebratory Delights: Festive Treats for Special Occasions 100

Balancing Indulgence and Moderation 100

Mindful Eating on Special Occasions: 101

Birthday Bash: Cake and Cupcake Delights.......................... 101

Diabetic-Friendly Chocolate Cake: 101

Mini Banana Cupcakes with Cream Cheese Frosting:............. 103

Holiday Extravaganza: Special Treats for Festive Seasons...... 106

Diabetic-Friendly Pumpkin Pie 106

Festive Berry Trifle 108

Conclusion 110

Introduction

Understanding Diabetes and Nutrition

What is Diabetes?

Living with diabetes can be challenging, but with the right knowledge and approach to nutrition, you can lead a fulfilling and healthy life. Let's start by understanding what diabetes is and its various types.

Diabetes is a chronic medical condition that affects how your body processes glucose, a type of sugar that serves as the primary source of energy for our cells. When we consume food, our bodies break down carbohydrates into glucose, which enters the bloodstream. In response, the pancreas releases insulin, a hormone that helps transport glucose from the bloodstream into our cells, where it can be used for energy.

In the case of diabetes, this process is disrupted. There are primarily three types of diabetes:

Type 1 Diabetes: This occurs when the body's immune system mistakenly attacks and destroys the insulin-producing cells in the pancreas. As a result, individuals with Type 1 diabetes have little to no insulin production and require regular insulin injections to manage their blood sugar levels effectively.

Example: Sarah was diagnosed with Type 1 diabetes at the age of 10. Since then, she has been diligently monitoring her blood sugar levels and administering insulin as prescribed by her doctor.

Type 2 Diabetes: This is the most common type of diabetes and usually develops later in life. In Type 2 diabetes, the body either doesn't produce enough insulin or becomes resistant to the effects of insulin, leading to elevated blood sugar levels.

Example: Michael was diagnosed with Type 2 diabetes in his 50s. He manages his condition through a combination of dietary changes, exercise, and oral medications.

Gestational Diabetes: This type occurs during pregnancy when hormonal changes can lead to insulin resistance. Most women with gestational diabetes return to normal blood sugar levels after childbirth. However, they are at a higher risk of developing Type 2 diabetes later in life.

Example: Jennifer was diagnosed with gestational diabetes during her pregnancy. She diligently followed her doctor's dietary recommendations and maintained regular check-ups to ensure a healthy pregnancy.

Section 2: The Importance of Nutrition in Diabetes Management

One of the most crucial aspects of managing diabetes is maintaining a well-balanced and nutritious diet. Proper nutrition plays a significant role in regulating blood sugar levels, managing weight, and reducing the risk of complications associated with diabetes.

Carbohydrates and Glycemic Index:

Carbohydrates have the most significant impact on blood sugar levels, so understanding how they affect your body is essential. The glycemic index (GI) is a scale that ranks carbohydrate-containing foods based on their effect on blood glucose levels. Foods with a high GI cause rapid spikes in blood sugar, while those with a low GI result in slower, more gradual increases.

Example: Choosing whole grains such as brown rice and quinoa over white rice can help maintain steadier blood sugar levels due to their lower GI.

Fiber: This is an essential component of a diabetes-friendly diet. It slows down the absorption of sugar, which can help prevent sharp spikes in blood glucose levels after meals.

Example: Adding more fiber-rich foods like vegetables, legumes, and whole fruits to your diet can positively impact blood sugar control.

<u>**Healthy Fats:**</u> Not all fats are created equal, and including healthy fats in your diet can be beneficial for diabetes management. Unsaturated fats, such as those found in avocados, nuts, and olive oil, can help improve insulin sensitivity.

Example: John incorporates a small handful of nuts into his afternoon snack to add healthy fats and protein to his diet, which helps him maintain stable blood sugar levels throughout the day.

Creating a Balanced Diabetes Meal Plan

Developing a well-balanced meal plan is the foundation of managing diabetes effectively. A balanced meal plan ensures that you get the necessary nutrients while keeping your blood sugar levels in check.

<u>**Portion Control:**</u> Controlling portion sizes is vital to managing blood sugar levels and body weight. Smaller, more frequent meals can help prevent large spikes in glucose levels.

Example: Maria uses a smaller plate to control her portion sizes and avoids going back for seconds to maintain a balanced diet.

Plate Method: The plate method is a practical way to create balanced meals. Fill half of your plate with non-starchy vegetables, a quarter with lean protein, and a quarter with whole grains or starchy vegetables.

Example: For dinner, Tom prepares a plate with grilled chicken, steamed broccoli, and a side of quinoa, following the plate method for a well-rounded meal.

Regular Meal Timings: Establishing regular meal timings can help regulate blood sugar levels and prevent extreme fluctuations.

Example: Emily sets alarms on her phone to remind her to eat at consistent intervals, ensuring she doesn't skip meals or go too long between eating.

Smart Snacking for Stable Blood Sugar Levels

Snacking can be an essential part of diabetes management, especially for those on insulin or medications that may cause hypoglycemia (low blood sugar). Smart snacking involves choosing nutrient-dense foods that won't cause drastic changes in blood glucose levels.

Protein-Packed Snacks: Protein can help stabilize blood sugar levels and keep you feeling full for longer. Opt for snacks that include lean protein sources.

Example: For an afternoon snack, Sarah enjoys Greek yogurt with a sprinkle of nuts and berries, a delicious and protein-rich option.

Avoiding Processed Sugars: Steer clear of snacks with added sugars or refined carbohydrates, as they can cause rapid spikes in blood sugar levels.

Example: Instead of sugary cookies, Michael snacks on apple slices with a tablespoon of natural peanut butter for a satisfying and blood sugar-friendly treat.

Pre-Portioned Snacks: Pre-portioned snacks help you control the number of carbohydrates you consume, making it easier to manage your blood sugar levels.

Example: Jennifer prepares individual snack bags filled with baby carrots, cucumber slices, and hummus, making it convenient to grab a healthy snack on the go.

Navigating Diabetic Dietary Requirements

Living with diabetes requires careful attention to your dietary choices. Understanding how different foods affect your blood sugar levels and learning to navigate diabetic dietary requirements are essential for managing this condition effectively. In this chapter, we will delve into the key aspects of diabetic dietary requirements and provide practical examples to help you make informed food choices.

Balancing Carbohydrates for Blood Sugar Control

Carbohydrates have the most significant impact on blood sugar levels, making them a crucial factor in diabetic dietary management. Learning to balance your carbohydrate intake is essential for maintaining stable blood glucose levels.

Counting Carbohydrates: One approach to managing carbohydrates is carbohydrate counting. This involves tracking the total amount of carbohydrates you consume and distributing them evenly throughout the day to prevent sharp spikes or drops in blood sugar.

Example: Before lunch, Mark checks the nutrition label on his bread to see that one slice contains 15 grams of carbohydrates. He decides to have two slices, equaling 30 grams of carbohydrates, for a well-distributed carbohydrate intake.

Glycemic Index and Load: Understanding the glycemic index (GI) and glycemic load (GL) of foods can help you choose carbohydrates that have a gentler impact on blood sugar levels. Low-GI foods cause slower and more gradual increases in blood sugar compared to high-GI foods.

Example: Emily swaps her usual white rice for quinoa, which has a lower GI, to help prevent sudden spikes in her blood sugar after meals.

High-Fiber Carbohydrates: Incorporating high-fiber carbohydrates into your diet can help slow down the absorption of sugar and improve blood sugar control.

Example: For breakfast, Sarah chooses oatmeal with added berries and chia seeds, providing both fiber and essential nutrients for a balanced start to her day.

The Role of Protein in Diabetes Management

Protein is an important nutrient that plays a significant role in diabetes management. It can help stabilize blood sugar levels and promote satiety, making it an excellent addition to your meals and snacks.

Lean Protein Sources: Opt for lean protein sources to avoid unnecessary saturated fats. Some examples of lean protein sources include skinless chicken, turkey, fish, tofu, and legumes.

Example: For dinner, Michael grills a piece of salmon and serves it with a side of steamed vegetables and a small portion of quinoa for a balanced and protein-rich meal.

Protein-Packed Snacks: Including protein in your snacks can help prevent blood sugar spikes between meals. Consider pairing protein with a small amount of carbohydrates to maintain steady glucose levels.

Example: Maria snacks on a handful of almonds and a few whole-grain crackers, combining protein and fiber to keep her blood sugar stable during the afternoon.

Managing Fats Wisely

Fats are an essential part of a diabetic diet, but not all fats are created equal. Understanding the different types of fats and making wise choices is crucial for maintaining heart health and overall well-being.

Choosing Healthy Fats: Opt for unsaturated fats, such as those found in avocados, nuts, seeds, and olive oil. These fats can help improve insulin sensitivity and support cardiovascular health.

Example: Jennifer prepares a salad with mixed greens, cherry tomatoes, avocado slices, and a drizzle of olive oil as a nutritious and diabetes-friendly lunch.

<u>Limiting Saturated and Trans Fats:</u> Reduce your intake of saturated and trans fats, commonly found in processed foods, fried items, and fatty cuts of meat. These fats can contribute to insulin resistance and increase the risk of heart disease.

Example: John replaces his usual fried snacks with baked versions, reducing his intake of unhealthy fats and making a positive impact on his blood sugar and heart health.

Monitoring Sodium Intake for Blood Pressure Control

People with diabetes are at an increased risk of developing hypertension (high blood pressure), which can further complicate the management of the condition. Monitoring sodium intake is crucial for blood pressure control and overall cardiovascular health.

<u>Reading Nutrition Labels</u>: Pay attention to the sodium content listed on nutrition labels to make informed choices about the foods you consume.

Example: Tom checks the sodium content on a can of soup before purchasing it, opting for a reduced-sodium version to support his blood pressure management.

<u>Cooking with Herbs and Spices:</u> Instead of relying on salt for flavoring, experiment with herbs and spices to enhance the taste of your meals without adding unnecessary sodium.

Example: Emily prepares a chicken stir-fry using a blend of garlic, ginger, and black pepper, adding a burst of flavor without relying on excess salt.

Smart Snacking for Stable Blood Sugar Levels

Snacking plays a crucial role in managing blood sugar levels for individuals living with diabetes. Strategic and thoughtful snacking can help prevent extreme fluctuations in glucose levels and provide sustained energy throughout the day. In this chapter, we will explore the art of smart snacking and offer specific examples to guide you in making delicious and blood sugar-friendly choices.

The Role of Snacks in Diabetes Management

Snacks can be an essential tool in diabetes management, especially for those taking insulin or medications that may cause hypoglycemia (low blood sugar). Understanding the role of snacks and their impact on blood sugar levels is vital for making informed choices.

Preventing Blood Sugar Dips: Well-planned snacks can help prevent blood sugar levels from dropping too low between meals, avoiding symptoms of hypoglycemia, such as shakiness, dizziness, and confusion.

Example: Jennifer keeps a small bag of mixed nuts in her purse to snack on when she feels her blood sugar levels dropping.

Managing Portion Sizes: Controlling portion sizes is crucial when snacking to avoid consuming excessive carbohydrates or calories, which can lead to blood sugar spikes.

Example: Tom divides a large bag of baby carrots into individual portion-sized containers to have a ready-to-go and diabetes-friendly snack.

Protein-Packed Snacks for Sustained Energy

Incorporating protein into your snacks is an excellent way to maintain stable blood sugar levels and provide long-lasting energy. Protein slows down the absorption of carbohydrates, preventing rapid spikes in blood sugar.

Greek Yogurt with Berries: A classic and delicious protein-packed snack option is Greek yogurt topped with fresh berries. Greek yogurt is rich in protein and calcium, while berries provide natural sweetness and fiber.

Example: Emily enjoys a bowl of Greek yogurt with a handful of blueberries and a sprinkle of almonds as an afternoon pick-me-up.

Hard-Boiled Eggs: Hard-boiled eggs are convenient and portable snacks that offer a good balance of protein and healthy fats, making them an excellent choice for steady energy.

Example: Michael prepares a batch of hard-boiled eggs at the beginning of the week to have a quick and satisfying snack option readily available.

Nuts and Seeds for Satiety

Nuts and seeds are nutrient-dense snacks that provide a combination of protein, healthy fats, and fiber. They help keep you feeling full and satisfied between meals.

Almonds: Almonds are a popular choice for a diabetes-friendly snack due to their rich content of healthy monounsaturated fats and protein.

Example: Sarah carries a small container of almonds in her bag to snack on when she's on the go and needs a quick and nutritious bite.

Chia Seed Pudding: Chia seed pudding is a delightful and versatile snack that can be prepared in advance and customized with various toppings.

Example: John prepares a batch of chia seed pudding with unsweetened almond milk and tops it with a few slices of fresh fruit for a delicious and filling snack.

Incorporating Fruits and Vegetables

Fruits and vegetables are excellent choices for snacking as they provide essential vitamins, minerals, and fiber, while some are naturally low in carbohydrates.

Celery Sticks with Peanut Butter: Celery sticks paired with natural peanut butter offer a crunchy and satisfying snack that combines fiber and protein.

Example: Maria enjoys the combination of celery sticks and peanut butter as a light snack before her evening walk.

Sliced Cucumber with Hummus: Cucumber slices dipped in hummus make a refreshing and nutrient-rich snack option that is low in carbohydrates.

Example: Mark prepares a plate of cucumber slices with a side of hummus to enjoy during his afternoon break at work.

Avoiding Processed Sugars and Refined Carbohydrates

Steer clear of snacks high in added sugars and refined carbohydrates, as they can cause rapid spikes in blood sugar levels.

Dark Chocolate with Almonds: Opt for dark chocolate with a high cocoa content and a moderate amount of almonds for a decadent yet diabetes-friendly treat.

Example: Emily treats herself to a small piece of dark chocolate with a few almonds when she craves something sweet after dinner.

<u>Baked Sweet Potato Fries:</u> Making baked sweet potato fries at home allows you to control the amount of oil and seasoning, making them a healthier alternative to regular potato chips.

Example: Michael cuts sweet potatoes into thin strips, lightly tosses them in olive oil, and bakes them in the oven until crispy for a guilt-free snack.

Decadent Desserts without the Guilt

Living with diabetes doesn't mean you have to give up on enjoying delicious desserts. With a bit of creativity and some smart ingredient substitutions, you can indulge in decadent treats that won't send your blood sugar levels soaring. In this chapter, we'll explore a variety of mouthwatering dessert options that will satisfy your sweet tooth without compromising your health.

Embracing Natural Sweeteners

One of the key secrets to creating guilt-free desserts for diabetes management is the use of natural sweeteners. These alternatives to refined sugar can add sweetness to your treats without causing rapid spikes in blood sugar levels.

Stevia: Stevia is a natural sweetener derived from the leaves of the Stevia plant. It is a popular choice for individuals with diabetes due to its minimal impact on blood sugar.

Example: Emily uses stevia to sweeten her homemade lemonade and enjoys it on a warm summer afternoon without worrying about her blood sugar levels.

Monk Fruit: Monk fruit sweetener is extracted from monk fruit and contains no calories or carbohydrates, making it a suitable option for those looking to avoid sugar.

Example: Michael uses monk fruit sweetener to prepare a delicious fruit salad, enhancing the natural sweetness of the fruits without adding any additional sugar.

Incorporating Whole Grains

Whole grains are a great addition to diabetes-friendly desserts as they provide fiber, which can slow down the absorption of sugar and help stabilize blood glucose levels.

Oatmeal Cookies: Swap traditional flour for oat flour when making cookies to add fiber and reduce the overall carbohydrate content.

Example: Sarah bakes oatmeal raisin cookies using oat flour, which results in a chewy and satisfying treat that won't cause drastic fluctuations in her blood sugar levels.

Quinoa Pudding: Quinoa is a protein-rich whole grain that can be used as a base for a creamy and delightful pudding.

Example: John prepares quinoa pudding with unsweetened almond milk, cinnamon, and a touch of vanilla extract, creating a luscious dessert that is kind to his blood sugar.

Exploring Fruit-Based Desserts

Fruits offer natural sweetness and essential vitamins, making them an excellent foundation for guilt-free desserts.

Berry Parfait: Layering fresh berries with Greek yogurt and a sprinkle of nuts creates a beautiful and healthy parfait with the perfect balance of sweetness and protein.

Example: Maria assembles a berry parfait with strawberries, blueberries, and raspberries, making it a delightful and visually appealing dessert.

Baked Apples: Baking apples with a sprinkle of cinnamon and a drizzle of honey or maple syrup results in a warm and comforting treat that feels indulgent without causing a sugar spike.

Example: Tom bakes apples stuffed with a mixture of chopped nuts, cinnamon, and a touch of honey, creating a flavorful dessert that he enjoys with a dollop of Greek yogurt.

Utilizing Nut Flours and Meals

Nut flours and meals are excellent alternatives to traditional refined flours, as they are lower in carbohydrates and provide healthy fats and protein.

Almond Flour Brownies: Replace regular flour with almond flour when making brownies to create a moist and fudgy dessert with a lower glycemic impact.

Example: Emily bakes almond flour brownies and shares them with her friends, who can't believe they are diabetes-friendly due to their rich texture and flavor.

Coconut Flour Cake: Coconut flour is a versatile option for baking, and when used in cakes, it results in a moist and tender crumb.

Example: Michael bakes a coconut flour lemon cake for a family gathering, impressing everyone with the light and citrusy flavors.

Frozen Delights

Frozen desserts can be a refreshing treat, especially during warmer months, and there are plenty of diabetes-friendly options to explore.

Sugar-Free Sorbet: Making sorbet at home with fresh fruit and natural sweeteners provides a refreshing and naturally sweet dessert without added sugars.

Example: Sarah prepares a watermelon sorbet using fresh watermelon, lime juice, and a touch of stevia, offering a guilt-free and cooling treat.

<u>Yogurt Popsicles:</u> Creating popsicles with Greek yogurt and blended fruit is a fun and healthy way to enjoy frozen desserts.

Example: John blends Greek yogurt with mixed berries and a drizzle of honey, pours the mixture into popsicle molds, and freezes them for a delicious and satisfying dessert.

Fruity Indulgences: Berry Bliss

For those with a sweet tooth and diabetes, berries are a delightful and guilt-free indulgence. Packed with natural sweetness and essential nutrients, these tiny powerhouses of flavor make for a perfect addition to diabetes-friendly desserts. In this chapter, we'll explore the wonderful world of berry-inspired treats that will leave your taste buds dancing with joy.

Nutritional Benefits of Berries

Berries are not only delicious but also highly nutritious. Incorporating these vibrant fruits into your diet offers a range of health benefits, making them a delightful addition to your diabetes management plan.

Rich in Antioxidants: Berries are loaded with antioxidants, such as vitamin C and anthocyanins, which help combat oxidative stress and inflammation in the body.

Example: Strawberries, blueberries, and raspberries are excellent sources of antioxidants, contributing to overall well-being.

Low in Sugar and Carbohydrates: Compared to other fruits, berries are relatively low in sugar and carbohydrates, making them a diabetes-friendly choice.

Example: Blackberries contain just 7 grams of net carbs per 100 grams, making them a suitable option for those managing their blood sugar levels.

Fresh Berry Delights

Enjoying fresh berries on their own or paired with other ingredients creates simple yet satisfying desserts that celebrate the natural sweetness of these fruits.

Mixed Berry Salad: Tossing together a medley of fresh berries creates a colorful and refreshing berry salad that can be enjoyed as a light dessert or a snack.

Example: Emily prepares a berry salad with a mix of strawberries, blueberries, and blackberries, adding a splash of lime juice for a zesty twist.

Berries and Greek Yogurt: Pairing fresh berries with Greek yogurt provides a creamy and protein-rich dessert that is both satisfying and nutritious.

Example: Michael layers Greek yogurt with sliced strawberries and a drizzle of honey for a delightful and guilt-free parfait.

Berry-licious Smoothies

Smoothies are a fantastic way to blend different berries with other ingredients to create a wholesome and flavorful treat.

Triple Berry Smoothie: Blending strawberries, blueberries, and raspberries with unsweetened almond milk creates a delightful triple berry smoothie that bursts with fruity goodness.

Example: Sarah enjoys a triple berry smoothie for breakfast, adding a handful of spinach for an extra dose of nutrients.

<u>**Mixed Berry Green Smoothie:**</u> Adding a handful of berries to a green smoothie enhances the flavor and brings natural sweetness without the need for added sugars.

Example: John blends spinach, kale, a scoop of protein powder, and a handful of mixed berries for a nutritious and energizing green smoothie.

Baked Berry Treats

Incorporating berries into baked goods provides a burst of flavor and a touch of natural sweetness, making them a delightful indulgence.

<u>**Blueberry Almond Muffins:**</u> Adding fresh blueberries and almond flour to muffins results in a moist and flavorful treat that won't cause sharp spikes in blood sugar levels.

Example: Maria bakes a batch of blueberry almond muffins for a weekend brunch, sharing the joy of guilt-free indulgence with her friends.

Raspberry Chia Seed Jam: Preparing chia seed jam with raspberries and a touch of natural sweetener offers a spreadable delight without added sugars.

Example: Tom spreads raspberry chia seed jam on whole-grain toast for a delicious and nutritious breakfast option.

Frozen Berry Delicacies

Freezing berries allows you to create delightful frozen treats that are perfect for hot summer days.

Mixed Berry Sorbet: Blending a mix of berries with a splash of lemon juice and a natural sweetener creates a refreshing and sugar-conscious sorbet.

Example: Emily makes a mixed berry sorbet using stevia as a sweetener, enjoying it as a cooling dessert on a warm evening.

Strawberry Frozen Yogurt: Combining frozen strawberries with Greek yogurt and a drizzle of honey creates a creamy and tangy frozen yogurt without added sugars.

Example: Michael prepares strawberry frozen yogurt for his family, who can't believe it's both diabetes-friendly and utterly delicious.

Nutty Delights: Irresistible Treats with Nuts

Nuts are a treasure trove of flavor and nutrition, making them a perfect addition to diabetes-friendly desserts. Packed with healthy fats, protein, and essential vitamins, nuts offer a delightful crunch and a touch of indulgence to your sweet creations. In this chapter, we'll explore the world of nutty delights, showcasing irresistible treats that will satisfy your cravings without compromising your blood sugar management.

The Nutritional Benefits of Nuts

Nuts are not only delicious but also highly nutritious. Understanding their health benefits can help you appreciate these little powerhouses even more.

Healthy Fats: Nuts are rich in heart-healthy monounsaturated and polyunsaturated fats, which can help improve insulin sensitivity and support cardiovascular health.

Example: Almonds, walnuts, and pistachios are excellent sources of healthy fats, making them a delightful addition to diabetes-friendly desserts.

Protein: Nuts provide a good dose of plant-based protein, which can help keep you feeling full and satisfied.

Example: Adding a sprinkle of nuts to your desserts not only adds texture but also contributes to the overall protein content of the treat.

Nutty Toppings and Mix-ins

Incorporating nuts as toppings or mix-ins in your desserts elevates the flavor and adds a delightful crunch to your creations.

Nutty Granola: Creating homemade granola with a mix of nuts, seeds, and whole grains offers a nutritious topping for yogurt, smoothies, or fruit bowls.

Example: Emily bakes a batch of nutty granola with almonds, pecans, and pumpkin seeds, enjoying it as a delightful and fiber-rich topping for her breakfast parfaits.

Nut Butter Swirls: Drizzling nut butter, such as almond or peanut butter, over your desserts adds a creamy and nutty touch without the need for added sugars.

Example: Michael swirls almond butter into his banana nice cream, creating a luscious and satisfying treat with a burst of nutty goodness.

Nutty Energy Bites

Energy bites are convenient and nutritious treats that combine the goodness of nuts with other wholesome ingredients.

Almond Date Energy Bites: Blending almonds and dates with a touch of cinnamon and vanilla creates a nutritious and naturally sweetened energy bite.

Example: Sarah prepares almond date energy bites, which she enjoys as a quick pick-me-up when she needs a burst of energy during the day.

Hazelnut Cocoa Bites: Combining hazelnuts, cocoa powder, and unsweetened shredded coconut creates a delectable and energy-packed treat with a hint of chocolatey flavor.

Example: John rolls hazelnut cocoa bites in a dusting of cocoa powder, making them an irresistible and guilt-free after-dinner dessert.

Nuts in Baked Treats

Incorporating nuts into your baked goods adds depth of flavor and texture to your diabetes-friendly desserts.

Pecan Pie Bars: Creating pecan pie bars with a nutty crust and a reduced-sugar filling offers all the delightful flavors of the classic dessert without the excess sugar.

Example: Maria bakes pecan pie bars for a family gathering, sharing the joy of nutty indulgence with her loved ones.

<u>**Walnut Banana Bread**</u>: Adding chopped walnuts to banana bread brings an extra layer of flavor and crunch to this classic treat.

Example: Tom bakes a loaf of walnut banana bread, which he enjoys as a satisfying and wholesome breakfast or a delightful afternoon snack.

Nutty Frozen Delicacies

Nuts can be incorporated into frozen desserts to create delectable treats for hot summer days.

<u>**Pistachio Ice Cream:**</u> Using unsweetened pistachio butter or ground pistachios in homemade ice cream results in a creamy and flavorful treat without added sugars.

Example: Emily prepares pistachio ice cream using a mixture of pistachio butter and coconut milk, indulging in a delightful frozen dessert without worries about her blood sugar.

<u>Nutty Ice Pops:</u> Blending nuts with frozen fruit and a touch of yogurt or milk creates nutty ice pops that are both refreshing and satisfying.

Example: Michael blends mixed nuts with frozen strawberries and a splash of almond milk to make nutty ice pops that are perfect for cooling off on a warm day.

Chocolate Lover's Paradise: Sinless Cocoa Creations

For chocolate lovers with diabetes, the thought of indulging in sweet cocoa treats might seem like an impossible dream. However, with the right approach and smart ingredient choices, you can enjoy sinless cocoa creations that won't wreak havoc on your blood sugar levels. In this chapter, we'll dive into the realm of chocolate-inspired desserts that will delight your taste buds without compromising your health.

The Health Benefits of Dark Chocolate

Dark chocolate, with a high cocoa content and minimal added sugars, offers several health benefits that make it a perfect choice for diabetes-friendly desserts.

Rich in Antioxidants: Dark chocolate is packed with antioxidants, such as flavonoids, which help neutralize harmful free radicals in the body.

Example: Opting for dark chocolate with a cocoa content of at least 70% ensures you're reaping the full antioxidant benefits.

Improved Insulin Sensitivity: Studies suggest that dark chocolate may improve insulin sensitivity, potentially benefiting those with diabetes.

Example: Incorporating small amounts of dark chocolate into your desserts can be a delightful way to enjoy its potential health benefits.

Mindful Chocolate Choices

When selecting chocolate for your desserts, it's essential to be mindful of its cocoa content and added sugar levels.

Choosing High-Cocoa Dark Chocolate: Opt for dark chocolate with a cocoa content of 70% or higher to minimize the sugar content and maximize the health benefits.

Example: Emily uses 80% dark chocolate in her cocoa creations, appreciating the deep and rich flavor it brings to her desserts.

<u>**Unsweetened Cocoa Powder:**</u> Using unsweetened cocoa powder in your recipes allows you to control the amount of sugar in your desserts.

Example: Michael prepares a batch of unsweetened cocoa powder brownies, enjoying the intense chocolate flavor without excessive sweetness.

Guilt-Free Chocolate Treats

Creating sinless cocoa creations with diabetes-friendly ingredients is both satisfying and delicious.

<u>**Dark Chocolate Avocado Mousse:**</u> Blending ripe avocado with melted dark chocolate and a touch of sweetener creates a creamy and rich chocolate mousse.

Example: Sarah prepares dark chocolate avocado mousse for a dinner party, impressing her guests with the velvety texture and delightful taste.

<u>**Chocolate-Dipped Strawberries:**</u> Dipping fresh strawberries in melted dark chocolate results in a simple yet elegant dessert that satisfies chocolate cravings.

Example: Tom prepares a platter of chocolate-dipped strawberries for a romantic evening, enjoying the delightful combination of sweet and tart flavors.

Creative Cocoa Confections

Incorporating cocoa into your desserts can lead to creative and sinless delights that cater to your chocolate cravings.

<u>**Cocoa Nib Energy Bars:**</u> Mixing cocoa nibs with nuts, seeds, and dates creates a nutritious and energy-packed bar with a delightful chocolate crunch.

Example: Maria prepares cocoa nib energy bars to take with her on hikes, enjoying the natural sweetness and sustained energy they provide.

<u>**Chocolate Chia Pudding:**</u> Combining chia seeds with unsweetened cocoa powder and almond milk creates a luscious and fiber-rich chocolate chia pudding.

Example: John prepares chocolate chia pudding for a quick and nourishing breakfast, savoring the creamy texture and chocolaty goodness.

Frozen Chocolate Delights

Frozen chocolate treats offer a refreshing way to indulge in cocoa goodness, especially during warm weather.

<u>**Chocolate Banana Nice Cream:**</u> Blending frozen bananas with unsweetened cocoa powder results in a guilt-free and creamy chocolate nice cream.

Example: Emily whips up a batch of chocolate banana nice cream for her family, who can't believe it's both diabetes-friendly and decadent.

<u>**Chocolate Almond Milkshake:**</u> Blending unsweetened almond milk with dark chocolate and a dash of

vanilla extract creates a delightful and cooling chocolate milkshake.

Example: Michael enjoys a chocolate almond milkshake on a hot summer day, appreciating the satisfying flavors without excessive sugars.

Wholesome Baked Goods: Cakes, Muffins & More

Wholesome baked goods can be a delightful addition to a diabetes-friendly diet, offering a mix of flavors and textures that cater to your sweet cravings without causing drastic spikes in blood sugar levels. In this chapter, we'll explore a variety of nutritious and delicious baked goods, including cakes, muffins, and more, that you and your family can enjoy guilt-free. These recipes are designed to be friendly to both adults and kids, providing a balanced and satisfying treat for all.

Smart Ingredient Swaps for Baked Goods

Making smart ingredient substitutions in baked goods can significantly reduce the sugar and carbohydrate content while maintaining the flavor and texture you love.

Whole Grain Flours: Replace refined flours with whole grain flours, such as whole wheat or almond flour, to add fiber and nutrients to your baked treats.

Example Recipe: Whole Wheat Banana Nut Muffins Serving Portions: Adults - 1 muffin, Kids - 1/2 muffin

Ingredients:

- 1 cup whole wheat flour
- 1/2 cup chopped nuts (walnuts or almonds)
- 1 teaspoon baking powder
- 1/2 teaspoon baking soda
- 1/4 teaspoon salt
- 2 ripe bananas, mashed
- 1/3 cup unsweetened applesauce
- 1/4 cup honey or maple syrup
- 1/4 cup unsweetened almond milk
- 1 teaspoon vanilla extract

Instructions:

1. Preheat your oven to 350°F (175°C). Line a muffin tin with paper liners or grease it lightly.
2. In a large bowl, whisk together the whole wheat flour, chopped nuts, baking powder, baking soda, and salt.

3. In a separate bowl, mix the mashed bananas, applesauce, honey or maple syrup, almond milk, and vanilla extract.

4. Pour the wet ingredients into the dry ingredients and stir until just combined.

5. Divide the batter evenly among the muffin cups.

6. Bake for 18-20 minutes or until a toothpick inserted in the center comes out clean.

7. Allow the muffins to cool for a few minutes before serving.

Natural Sweeteners:

Use natural sweeteners, such as honey, maple syrup, or stevia, in place of refined sugars to add sweetness without causing rapid blood sugar spikes.

Example Recipe: Maple Cinnamon Carrot Cake
Serving Portions: Adults - 1 slice, Kids - 1/2 slice

Ingredients:

- 1 ½ cups whole wheat flour
- 2 teaspoons baking powder

- ½ teaspoon baking soda
- ¼ teaspoon salt
- 1 teaspoon ground cinnamon
- ½ cup unsweetened applesauce
- 1/3 cup pure maple syrup
- ¼ cup coconut oil, melted
- 2 large eggs
- 1 teaspoon vanilla extract
- 1 ½ cups grated carrots

Instructions:

1. Preheat your oven to 350°F (175°C). Grease a cake pan or line it with parchment paper.
2. In a large bowl, whisk together the whole wheat flour, baking powder, baking soda, salt, and ground cinnamon.
3. In a separate bowl, mix the applesauce, maple syrup, melted coconut oil, eggs, and vanilla extract.
4. Pour the wet ingredients into the dry ingredients and stir until well combined.
5. Fold in the grated carrots.
6. Pour the batter into the prepared cake pan.

7. Bake for 25-30 minutes or until a toothpick inserted in the center comes out clean.

8. Allow the cake to cool in the pan for 10 minutes before transferring it to a wire rack to cool completely.

Muffins and Cupcakes

Muffins and cupcakes can be versatile and satisfying baked treats, and with some thoughtful ingredient choices, they become diabetes-friendly delights.

Berry Oat Muffins

Serving Portions: Adults - 1 muffin, Kids - 1/2 muffin

Ingredients:

- 1 cup rolled oats
- 1 cup whole wheat flour
- 1 teaspoon baking powder
- 1/2 teaspoon baking soda
- 1/4 teaspoon salt
- 1/2 cup unsweetened applesauce

- 1/4 cup honey or agave nectar
- 1/4 cup unsweetened almond milk
- 2 tablespoons coconut oil, melted
- 1 large egg
- 1 teaspoon vanilla extract
- 1 cup fresh or frozen mixed berries (blueberries, raspberries, strawberries)

<u>Instructions:</u>

1. Preheat your oven to 375°F (190°C). Line a muffin tin with paper liners or grease it lightly.
2. In a blender or food processor, pulse the rolled oats until they resemble a coarse flour.
3. In a large bowl, whisk together the oat flour, whole wheat flour, baking powder, baking soda, and salt.
4. In a separate bowl, mix the applesauce, honey or agave nectar, almond milk, melted coconut oil, egg, and vanilla extract.

5. Pour the wet ingredients into the dry ingredients and stir until just combined.
6. Gently fold in the mixed berries.
7. Divide the batter evenly among the muffin cups.
8. Bake for 18-20 minutes or until a toothpick inserted in the center comes out clean.
9. Allow the muffins to cool for a few minutes before serving.

Chocolate Zucchini Cupcakes with Greek Yogurt Frosting

Serving Portions: Adults - 1 cupcake, Kids - 1/2 cupcake

Ingredients:

- 1 cup whole wheat flour
- 1/4 cup unsweetened cocoa powder
- 1 teaspoon baking powder
- 1/2 teaspoon baking soda
- 1/4 teaspoon salt
- 1/2 cup unsweetened applesauce
- 1/4 cup honey or maple syrup

- 1/4 cup coconut oil, melted
- 1 large egg
- 1 teaspoon vanilla extract
- 1 cup grated zucchini, squeezed to remove excess moisture
- 1/2 cup plain Greek yogurt
- 1 tablespoon honey
- 1/2 teaspoon vanilla extract

Instructions:

1. Preheat your oven to 350°F (175°C). Line a cupcake tin with paper liners or grease it lightly.
2. In a large bowl, whisk together the whole wheat flour, cocoa powder, baking powder, baking soda, and salt.
3. In a separate bowl, mix the applesauce, honey or maple syrup, melted coconut oil, egg, and vanilla extract.
4. Pour the wet ingredients into the dry ingredients and stir until well combined.
5. Fold in the grated zucchini.

6. Divide the batter evenly among the cupcake cups.

7. Bake for 18-20 minutes or until a toothpick inserted in the center comes out clean.

8. Allow the cupcakes to cool completely before frosting.

9. For the Greek yogurt frosting, whisk together the plain Greek yogurt, honey, and vanilla extract until smooth. Spread the frosting on the cooled cupcakes.

Wholesome Cakes

Celebratory cakes can still be a part of your diabetes-conscious lifestyle with these nutritious and delicious options.

Lemon Poppy Seed Cake: Serving Portions: Adults - 1 slice, Kids - 1/2 slice

Ingredients:

- 1 1/2 cups whole wheat flour
- 1/2 cup almond flour
- 2 teaspoons baking powder

- 1/2 teaspoon baking soda
- 1/4 teaspoon salt
- 1/2 cup unsweetened applesauce
- 1/4 cup honey or agave nectar
- 1/4 cup coconut oil, melted
- 1/2 cup plain Greek yogurt
- 1 large egg
- 1 tablespoon lemon zest
- 1/4 cup fresh lemon juice
- 1 tablespoon poppy seeds

Instructions:

1. Preheat your oven to 350°F (175°C). Grease a cake pan or line it with parchment paper.

2. In a large bowl, whisk together the whole wheat flour, almond flour, baking powder, baking soda, and salt.

3. In a separate bowl, mix the applesauce, honey or agave nectar, melted coconut oil, Greek yogurt, egg, lemon zest, and lemon juice.

4. Pour the wet ingredients into the dry ingredients and stir until well combined.

5. Fold in the poppy seeds.

6. Pour the batter into the prepared cake pan.

7. Bake for 25-30 minutes or until a toothpick inserted in the center comes out clean.

8. Allow the cake to cool in the pan for 10 minutes before transferring it to a wire rack to cool completely.

Apple Cinnamon Coffee Cake: Serving Portions: Adults - 1 slice, Kids - 1/2 slice

Ingredients:

- 1 1/2 cups whole wheat flour
- 1 teaspoon baking powder
- 1/2 teaspoon baking soda
- 1/4 teaspoon salt
- 1 teaspoon ground cinnamon
- 1/2 cup unsweetened applesauce
- 1/4 cup honey or maple syrup
- 1/4 cup coconut oil, melted
- 1/2 cup plain Greek yogurt

- 1 large egg
- 1 teaspoon vanilla extract
- 1 large apple, peeled and chopped
- 2 tablespoons chopped walnuts or almonds

Instructions:

1. Preheat your oven to 350°F (175°C). Grease a cake pan or line it with parchment paper.
2. In a large bowl, whisk together the whole wheat flour, baking powder, baking soda, salt, and ground cinnamon.
3. In a separate bowl, mix the applesauce, honey or maple syrup, melted coconut oil, Greek yogurt, egg, and vanilla extract.
4. Pour the wet ingredients into the dry ingredients and stir until well combined.
5. Fold in the chopped apple and chopped nuts.
6. Pour the batter into the prepared cake pan.
7. Bake for 25-30 minutes or until a toothpick inserted in the center comes out clean.
8. Allow the cake to cool in the pan for 10 minutes before transferring it to a wire rack to cool completely.

Frozen Pleasures: Diabetic-Friendly Ice Creams

Frozen pleasures are not off-limits for individuals managing diabetes. With the right ingredients and mindful choices, you can indulge in delicious and diabetic-friendly ice creams that won't cause drastic spikes in your blood sugar levels. In this chapter, we'll explore a variety of frozen delights that will satisfy your sweet cravings and keep you cool on warm days. These recipes are designed to be friendly to both adults and kids, ensuring everyone can enjoy these frozen pleasures guilt-free.

The Quest for Diabetic-Friendly Ice Creams

Finding or creating diabetic-friendly ice creams can be a delightful journey of exploration and taste.

Low-Sugar and No-Sugar Options:

Look for or create ice creams that use natural sweeteners or are entirely sugar-free to avoid rapid blood sugar spikes.

Nut-Based Ice Creams:

Choosing ice creams made with nuts or nut-based milks can provide a creamy texture and add healthy fats and protein to your treat.

Creamy Dairy-Free Delights

Dairy-free ice creams are a fantastic option for individuals with lactose intolerance or those looking to reduce their dairy intake.

Coconut Milk Vanilla Ice Cream:

Serving Portions: Adults - 1 scoop, Kids - 1/2 scoop

<u>Ingredients:</u>

- 2 cans (13.5 oz each) full-fat coconut milk
- 1/4 cup honey or agave nectar
- 1 tablespoon coconut oil, melted
- 1 tablespoon pure vanilla extract
- Pinch of salt

<u>**Instructions:**</u>

1. In a blender or food processor, combine the coconut milk, honey or agave nectar, melted coconut oil, vanilla extract, and salt.
2. Blend until smooth and well combined.
3. Pour the mixture into an ice cream maker and churn according to the manufacturer's instructions.
4. Transfer the churned ice cream into a container and freeze for an additional 2-3 hours to firm up.
5. Serve in bowls or cones, and enjoy the creamy and dairy-free delight.

Almond Chocolate Chip Ice Cream:

Serving Portions: Adults - 1 scoop, Kids - 1/2 scoop

<u>**Ingredients:**</u>

- 1 1/2 cups unsweetened almond milk
- 1/4 cup almond butter
- 1/4 cup honey or maple syrup
- 2 tablespoons unsweetened cocoa powder

- 1 teaspoon pure vanilla extract
- 1/4 cup sugar-free dark chocolate chips

<u>Instructions:</u>

1. In a blender or food processor, combine the almond milk, almond butter, honey or maple syrup, cocoa powder, and vanilla extract.
2. Blend until smooth and well combined.
3. Stir in the sugar-free dark chocolate chips.
4. Pour the mixture into an ice cream maker and churn according to the manufacturer's instructions.
5. Transfer the churned ice cream into a container and freeze for an additional 2-3 hours to firm up.
6. Scoop the almond chocolate chip ice cream into bowls or cones, and enjoy this nutty and chocolaty treat.

Classic Favorites, Redefined

Traditional ice cream flavors can be recreated with diabetic-friendly ingredients to bring joy to your taste buds.

Strawberry Banana Nice Cream:

Serving Portions: Adults - 1 scoop, Kids - 1/2 scoop

Ingredients:

- 2 large ripe bananas, peeled and sliced
- 1 cup frozen strawberries
- 1/4 cup unsweetened almond milk
- 1 teaspoon pure vanilla extract

Instructions:

1. In a blender or food processor, combine the sliced bananas, frozen strawberries, almond milk, and vanilla extract.
2. Blend until smooth and creamy.
3. Transfer the mixture into an airtight container and freeze for 2-3 hours to firm up.
4. Scoop the strawberry banana nice cream into bowls or cones, and enjoy the naturally sweet and fruity delight.

Mint Chocolate Avocado Ice Cream:

Serving Portions: Adults - 1 scoop, Kids - 1/2 scoop

Ingredients:

- 2 ripe avocados, peeled and pitted
- 1/4 cup honey or agave nectar
- 1/4 cup unsweetened almond milk
- 1 teaspoon pure peppermint extract
- 1/4 cup sugar-free dark chocolate chips

Instructions:

1. In a blender or food processor, combine the ripe avocados, honey or agave nectar, almond milk, and peppermint extract.
2. Blend until smooth and well combined.
3. Stir in the sugar-free dark chocolate chips.
4. Transfer the mixture into an airtight container and freeze for 2-3 hours to firm up.

5. Scoop the mint chocolate avocado ice cream into bowls or cones, and enjoy this refreshing and creamy treat.

Chapter 10:

No-Bake Delicacies: Quick and Easy Desserts

No-bake desserts are a lifesaver for those managing diabetes, offering quick and easy sweet indulgence without the need for baking. In this chapter, we'll explore a variety of delightful no-bake delicacies that are both delicious and diabetes-friendly. These recipes are designed to be friendly to both adults and kids, providing a hassle-free and satisfying treat for everyone to enjoy.

The Joys of No-Bake Desserts

No-bake desserts offer a range of benefits, from saving time in the kitchen to preserving the nutritional value of ingredients.

Quick and Convenient:

No-bake desserts can be whipped up in no time, making them perfect for satisfying sudden sweet cravings or unexpected guests.

<u>**Preserving Nutritional Value:**</u>

Without the need for baking, no-bake desserts retain the natural goodness and nutritional value of their ingredients.

<u>**Nutritious and Tasty Energy Balls**</u>

Energy balls are versatile and nutrient-packed treats that provide a quick and healthy pick-me-up.

Peanut Butter Oat Energy Balls

Serving Portions: Adults - 2 balls, Kids - 1 ball

<u>**Ingredients:**</u>

- 1 cup old-fashioned rolled oats
- 1/2 cup natural peanut butter
- 1/4 cup honey or maple syrup
- 1/4 cup ground flaxseed
- 1/4 cup mini dark chocolate chips
- 1 teaspoon pure vanilla extract

Instructions:

1. In a large bowl, combine the rolled oats, peanut butter, honey or maple syrup, ground flaxseed, mini dark chocolate chips, and vanilla extract.
2. Stir until well combined.
3. Take small portions of the mixture and roll them into bite-sized balls.
4. Place the energy balls on a parchment-lined tray and refrigerate for at least 30 minutes to set.
5. Store the energy balls in an airtight container in the refrigerator for up to one week.

Almond Date Energy Balls

Serving Portions: Adults - 2 balls, Kids - 1 ball

Ingredients:

- 1 cup raw almonds
- 1 cup pitted dates
- 1/4 cup unsweetened shredded coconut
- 1/4 cup almond butter

- 1 teaspoon pure almond extract

<u>Instructions:</u>

1. In a food processor, pulse the raw almonds until they resemble coarse crumbs.
2. Add the pitted dates, shredded coconut, almond butter, and almond extract to the food processor.
3. Process until the mixture comes together and forms a sticky dough.
4. Take small portions of the dough and roll them into bite-sized balls.
5. Place the almond date energy balls on a parchment-lined tray and refrigerate for at least 30 minutes to set.
6. Store the energy balls in an airtight container in the refrigerator for up to one week.

Delightful Chilled Puddings

No-bake puddings offer a creamy and indulgent dessert without the need for cooking.

Chia Seed Pudding:

Serving Portions: Adults - 1/2 cup, Kids - 1/4 cup

Ingredients:

- 1/4 cup chia seeds
- 1 cup unsweetened almond milk
- 1 tablespoon honey or agave nectar
- 1/2 teaspoon pure vanilla extract
- Fresh berries for topping

Instructions:

1. In a bowl, combine the chia seeds, almond milk, honey or agave nectar, and vanilla extract.
2. Stir well to ensure the chia seeds are evenly distributed.
3. Cover the bowl and refrigerate the mixture for at least 4 hours or preferably overnight.
4. Before serving, give the chia pudding a good stir to break up any clumps.

5. Divide the chia seed pudding into individual serving cups or bowls.

6. Top with fresh berries for added sweetness and nutrition.

Avocado Chocolate Pudding

Serving Portions: Adults - 1/2 cup, Kids - 1/4 cup

Ingredients:

- 2 ripe avocados, peeled and pitted
- 1/4 cup unsweetened cocoa powder
- 1/4 cup honey or maple syrup
- 1/4 cup unsweetened almond milk
- 1 teaspoon pure vanilla extract
- Pinch of salt

Instructions:

1. In a blender or food processor, combine the ripe avocados, cocoa powder, honey or maple syrup, almond milk, vanilla extract, and salt.

2. Blend until smooth and creamy.

3. Divide the avocado chocolate pudding into individual serving cups or bowls.

4. Refrigerate the pudding for at least 1 hour before serving.

5. Top with a sprinkle of cocoa powder or shaved dark chocolate for a delightful finish.

Refreshing Fruit Parfaits

Fruit parfaits offer a refreshing and visually appealing dessert that's easy to put together.

Mixed Berry Yogurt Parfait

Serving Portions: Adults - 1 cup, Kids - 1/2 cup

Ingredients:

- 1 cup plain Greek yogurt
- 1 tablespoon honey or agave nectar
- 1/2 cup fresh mixed berries (strawberries, blueberries, raspberries)
- 1/4 cup granola (look for low-sugar options)

<u>**Instructions:**</u>

In a small bowl, mix the plain Greek yogurt with honey or agave nectar to sweeten.

In individual serving glasses or bowls, layer the sweetened yogurt, fresh mixed berries, and granola.

Repeat the layers until you fill the glasses or bowls.

Top with a few extra berries and a sprinkle of granola for added texture.

Refrigerate the fruit parfait for at least 30 minutes before serving.

Tropical Fruit Coconut Parfait

Serving Portions: Adults - 1 cup, Kids - 1/2 cup

<u>**Ingredients:**</u>

- 1 cup coconut milk (canned or carton)
- 1 tablespoon honey or agave nectar
- 1/2 cup diced tropical fruits (mango, pineapple, kiwi)

- 2 tablespoons unsweetened shredded coconut

<u>Instructions</u>:

1. In a small bowl, mix the coconut milk with honey or agave nectar to sweeten.
2. In individual serving glasses or bowls, layer the sweetened coconut milk, diced tropical fruits, and shredded coconut.
3. Repeat the layers until you fill the glasses or bowls.
4. Top with a sprinkle of shredded coconut for a tropical touch.
5. Refrigerate the fruit coconut parfait for at least 30 minutes before serving.

Chapter 11:

Kid-Friendly Snacks: Fun and Healthy Bites

When managing diabetes, it's essential to provide wholesome and nutritious snacks for both adults and kids. In this chapter, we'll explore a variety of fun and healthy snacks that appeal to children's taste buds while supporting stable blood sugar levels. These snacks are not only delicious but also diabetes-friendly, making them perfect for satisfying hunger pangs and keeping energy levels up throughout the day.

The Importance of Kid-Friendly Snacks

Kid-friendly snacks play a crucial role in ensuring children maintain balanced nutrition while managing diabetes.

Keeping Energy Levels Stable

Well-balanced snacks help regulate blood sugar levels and keep energy levels steady, preventing sudden spikes and crashes.

Supporting Growth and Development:

Nutrient-dense snacks support healthy growth and development in children, providing essential vitamins and minerals.

Wholesome Fruit Treats

Fruits are nature's candy and make for fantastic kid-friendly snacks that are both nutritious and sweet.

Fruit Kabobs:

Serving Portions: Adults - 2 kabobs, Kids - 1 kabob

Ingredients:

- Assorted fruits (strawberries, grapes, pineapple, melon, etc.)
- Wooden or metal skewers

Instructions:

1. Wash and cut the fruits into bite-sized pieces.

2. Thread the fruit pieces onto the skewers, alternating colors and shapes to make them visually appealing.

3. Serve the fruit kabobs on a platter or individual plates.

Apple Sandwiches

Serving Portions: Adults - 1 sandwich, Kids - 1/2 sandwich

Ingredients:

- 1 apple, cored and sliced into rounds
- Nut butter (peanut butter, almond butter, etc.)
- Granola
- Raisins or dried cranberries

Instructions:

1. Spread nut butter on one apple round.

2. Sprinkle granola and raisins or dried cranberries on top.

3. Place another apple round on top to create an "apple sandwich."

4. Repeat with the remaining apple slices.

5. Serve the apple sandwiches on a plate or in individual snack containers.

Creative Veggie Delights

Getting kids to enjoy vegetables can be fun and rewarding with these creative and tasty snacks.

Veggie "Sushi" Rolls

Serving Portions: Adults - 4 rolls, Kids - 2 rolls

Ingredients:

- Large lettuce leaves (butter lettuce, romaine, or collard greens)
- Sliced veggies (cucumber, carrot, bell pepper, avocado, etc.)
- Hummus or Greek yogurt dip

Instructions:

1. Lay the lettuce leaves flat and spread a thin layer of hummus or Greek yogurt dip on each leaf.

2. Place the sliced veggies in the center of each leaf.

3. Roll up the lettuce leaves to create "sushi" rolls.

4. Slice each roll into bite-sized pieces.

5. Serve the veggie "sushi" rolls on a platter or in individual snack containers.

Veggie Rainbow Sticks

Serving Portions: Adults - 1 plate, Kids - 1/2 plate

Ingredients:

- Assorted colorful veggies (carrot sticks, cucumber slices, cherry tomatoes, bell pepper strips, etc.)
- Hummus or Greek yogurt dip

Instructions:

1. Arrange the colorful veggie sticks on a plate to resemble a rainbow.

2. Serve the veggie rainbow sticks with a side of hummus or Greek yogurt dip.

Protein-Packed Nibbles

Protein-rich snacks help keep hunger at bay and support healthy growth and development.

Cheese and Turkey Roll-Ups

Serving Portions: Adults - 4 roll-ups, Kids - 2 roll-ups

<u>Ingredients:</u>

- Sliced turkey or chicken breast
- Cheese slices (cheddar, Swiss, etc.)
- Mustard or a thin layer of cream cheese (optional)

<u>Instructions:</u>

1. Lay the turkey or chicken slices flat.
2. Place a cheese slice on top and add a thin layer of mustard or cream cheese if desired.
3. Roll up the turkey and cheese slices to create roll-ups.
4. Secure each roll-up with a toothpick if needed.

5. Serve the cheese and turkey roll-ups on a plate or in individual snack containers.

Chickpea Snack Mix:

Serving Portions: Adults - 1 cup, Kids - 1/2 cup

Ingredients:

- 1 can chickpeas (garbanzo beans), drained and rinsed
- 1 tablespoon olive oil
- 1 teaspoon ground cumin
- 1 teaspoon paprika
- 1/2 teaspoon garlic powder
- Salt and pepper to taste
- Assorted nuts and seeds (almonds, cashews, pumpkin seeds, etc.)
- Dried fruit (raisins, apricots, etc.)

Instructions:

1. Preheat the oven to 400°F (200°C).
2. In a bowl, toss the chickpeas with olive oil, ground cumin, paprika, garlic powder, salt, and pepper until well coated.

3. Spread the seasoned chickpeas on a baking sheet in a single layer.

4. Roast in the oven for 20-25 minutes or until crispy, shaking the pan occasionally for even cooking.

5. Remove the chickpeas from the oven and let them cool.

6. Mix the roasted chickpeas with assorted nuts, seeds, and dried fruit to create a protein-packed snack mix.

7. Serve the chickpea snack mix in individual snack containers or a bowl.

Comforting Classics: Diabetic Desserts with a Twist

Finding comfort in classic desserts while managing diabetes is possible with a little creativity and some diabetes-friendly ingredient swaps. In this chapter, we'll explore a range of familiar and comforting desserts that have been modified to fit into a diabetes-conscious lifestyle. These desserts are designed to bring a sense of nostalgia and joy without causing drastic spikes in blood sugar levels. Both adults and kids can savor these delightful twists on classic favorites.

Redefining All-Time Favorites

Classic desserts can be reimagined with diabetic-friendly ingredients, preserving their essence while making them suitable for your dietary needs.

Apple Crisp with Oat Topping:

Serving Portions: Adults - 1/2 cup, Kids - 1/4 cup

Ingredients:

- 4 cups sliced apples (a mix of Granny Smith and Honeycrisp)
- 1 tablespoon lemon juice
- 1 tablespoon honey or maple syrup
- 1/2 teaspoon ground cinnamon
- 1/4 cup rolled oats
- 1/4 cup almond flour
- 2 tablespoons chopped walnuts or pecans
- 2 tablespoons coconut oil, melted

Instructions:

1. Preheat your oven to 375°F (190°C). Grease a baking dish.
2. In a large bowl, toss the sliced apples with lemon juice, honey or maple syrup, and ground cinnamon.
3. In a separate bowl, mix the rolled oats, almond flour, chopped nuts, and melted coconut oil.
4. Place the apple mixture in the greased baking dish and spread the oat topping evenly over the apples.

5. Bake for 25-30 minutes or until the apples are tender and the topping is golden brown.

6. Allow the apple crisp to cool slightly before serving.

Crustless Pumpkin Pie

Serving Portions: Adults - 1 slice, Kids - 1/2 slice

Ingredients:

- 1 can (15 oz) pure pumpkin puree
- 1/2 cup unsweetened almond milk
- 1/4 cup honey or agave nectar
- 2 large eggs
- 1 teaspoon ground cinnamon
- 1/2 teaspoon ground ginger
- 1/4 teaspoon ground nutmeg
- 1/4 teaspoon salt
- Whipped coconut cream for topping (optional)

Instructions:

1. Preheat your oven to 350°F (175°C). Grease a pie dish.

2. In a large bowl, whisk together the pumpkin puree, almond milk, honey or agave nectar, eggs, ground cinnamon, ground ginger, ground nutmeg, and salt until well combined.

3. Pour the pumpkin mixture into the greased pie dish.

4. Bake for 40-45 minutes or until the center is set.

5. Allow the crustless pumpkin pie to cool completely before serving.

6. Top with whipped coconut cream for a delightful finishing touch.

Guilt-Free Chocolate Treats

Satisfy your chocolate cravings with these guilt-free desserts that won't wreak havoc on your blood sugar levels.

Chocolate Avocado Pudding

Serving Portions: Adults - 1/2 cup, Kids - 1/4 cup

Ingredients:

- 2 ripe avocados, peeled and pitted
- 1/4 cup unsweetened cocoa powder
- 1/4 cup honey or agave nectar
- 1/4 cup unsweetened almond milk
- 1 teaspoon pure vanilla extract
- Pinch of salt

Instructions:

1. In a blender or food processor, combine the ripe avocados, cocoa powder, honey or agave nectar, almond milk, vanilla extract, and salt.
2. Blend until smooth and creamy.
3. Divide the chocolate avocado pudding into individual serving cups or bowls.
4. Refrigerate the pudding for at least 1 hour before serving.
5. Top with a sprinkle of cocoa powder or shaved dark chocolate for an extra touch of indulgence.

Chocolate Chia Seed Pudding:

Serving Portions: Adults - 1/2 cup, Kids - 1/4 cup

Ingredients:

- 1/4 cup chia seeds
- 1 cup unsweetened almond milk
- 1/4 cup unsweetened cocoa powder
- 1/4 cup honey or agave nectar
- 1 teaspoon pure vanilla extract
- Pinch of salt

Instructions:

1. In a bowl, whisk together the chia seeds, almond milk, cocoa powder, honey or agave nectar, vanilla extract, and salt until well combined.
2. Cover the bowl and refrigerate the mixture for at least 4 hours or preferably overnight.
3. Before serving, give the chocolate chia seed pudding a good stir to break up any clumps.
4. Divide the pudding into individual serving cups or bowls.

5. Top with a dollop of whipped coconut cream if desired.

Healthier Twists on Childhood Favorites

Childhood favorites can be adapted to suit a diabetes-conscious lifestyle, bringing back fond memories with every bite.

Banana-Oat Cookies:

Serving Portions: Adults - 2 cookies, Kids - 1 cookie

<u>Ingredients:</u>

- 2 ripe bananas, mashed
- 1 1/2 cups old-fashioned rolled oats
- 1/4 cup almond butter
- 1/4 cup honey or maple syrup
- 1 teaspoon pure vanilla extract
- Pinch of salt
- Optional mix-ins: dark chocolate chips, chopped nuts, dried fruits

Instructions:

1. Preheat your oven to 350°F (175°C). Line a baking sheet with parchment paper.

2. In a large bowl, combine the mashed bananas, rolled oats, almond butter, honey or maple syrup, vanilla extract, and salt.

3. Mix until all the ingredients are well incorporated.

4. If desired, fold in your preferred mix-ins (dark chocolate chips, chopped nuts, dried fruits, etc.).

5. Scoop the cookie dough onto the prepared baking sheet, forming small cookie rounds.

6. Flatten the cookies slightly with the back of a spoon.

7. Bake for 12-15 minutes or until the cookies are lightly golden around the edges.

8. Allow the banana-oat cookies to cool on the baking sheet before transferring them to a wire rack to cool completely.

Yogurt Berry Parfaits:

Serving Portions: Adults - 1 cup, Kids - 1/2 cup

Ingredients:

- 2 cups plain Greek yogurt
- 2 tablespoons honey or agave nectar
- 1 teaspoon pure vanilla extract
- 1 cup mixed berries (strawberries, blueberries, raspberries)
- 1/4 cup granola (look for low-sugar options)

Instructions:

1. In a bowl, mix the plain Greek yogurt with honey or agave nectar and vanilla extract to sweeten.
2. In individual serving glasses or bowls, layer the sweetened yogurt, mixed berries, and granola.
3. Repeat the layers until you fill the glasses or bowls.
4. Top the yogurt berry parfaits with a few extra berries and a sprinkle of granola for added texture.

5. Refrigerate the parfaits for at least 30 minutes before serving.

International Flavors: Global Diabetic Dessert Recipes

Travel the world through desserts without leaving the comfort of your kitchen! In this chapter, we'll explore a diverse array of diabetic-friendly dessert recipes inspired by flavors from around the globe. These delightful treats are designed to bring the excitement of international cuisines to your diabetes-conscious lifestyle, satisfying your sweet cravings while keeping your blood sugar levels in check. Both adults and kids can embark on this delicious journey and savor the global flavors in each delectable bite.

Embracing the Richness of Asian Desserts

Asian desserts are known for their delicate flavors and use of unique ingredients that lend a touch of elegance to your sweet indulgence.

Mango Sticky Rice Pudding:

Serving Portions: Adults - 1/2 cup, Kids - 1/4 cup

<u>**Ingredients:**</u>

1 cup sticky rice (glutinous rice), soaked in water for 4 hours or overnight

1 1/2 cups coconut milk

1/4 cup honey or agave nectar

Pinch of salt

Fresh ripe mango slices for topping

<u>**Instructions:**</u>

1. Drain the soaked sticky rice and rinse it thoroughly.
2. In a saucepan, combine the sticky rice, coconut milk, honey or agave nectar, and salt.
3. Bring the mixture to a simmer over medium heat, stirring occasionally.
4. Reduce the heat to low and cover the saucepan. Let the rice cook for about 15-20 minutes or until tender and fully cooked.

5. Remove the saucepan from the heat and let the rice sit for 5 minutes to absorb any remaining liquid.

6. Serve the mango sticky rice pudding warm or at room temperature, topped with fresh mango slices.

Matcha Green Tea Mochi:

Serving Portions: Adults - 2 mochi, Kids - 1 mochi

Ingredients:

- 1 cup sweet rice flour (glutinous rice flour)
- 1/4 cup honey or agave nectar
- 2 teaspoons matcha green tea powder
- 1/2 cup water
- Cornstarch for dusting

Instructions:

1. In a microwave-safe bowl, mix the sweet rice flour, honey or agave nectar, matcha green tea powder, and water until well combined.

2. Cover the bowl with plastic wrap and microwave on high for 2 minutes.

3. Remove the bowl from the microwave and stir the mixture with a spatula.

4. Cover the bowl again and microwave for an additional 1 minute.

5. Transfer the mochi dough onto a surface lightly dusted with cornstarch.

6. Knead the mochi dough until it becomes smooth and pliable.

7. Divide the mochi dough into small portions and shape them into round or square pieces.

8. Serve the matcha green tea mochi immediately or store them in an airtight container in the refrigerator.

Celebrating the Flavors of the Mediterranean

The Mediterranean region offers a delightful array of desserts that are both light and satisfying, often featuring fruits and nuts.

Greek Yogurt with Honey and Pistachios:

Serving Portions: Adults - 1/2 cup, Kids - 1/4 cup

Ingredients:

- 2 cups plain Greek yogurt
- 2 tablespoons honey
- 1/4 cup chopped pistachios

Instructions:

1. In a bowl, sweeten the plain Greek yogurt with honey, mixing until well combined.
2. Divide the sweetened yogurt into individual serving cups or bowls.
3. Sprinkle the chopped pistachios on top of each serving.
4. Serve the Greek yogurt with honey and pistachios chilled for a refreshing treat.

Orange and Almond Cake (Gluten-Free)

Serving Portions: Adults - 1 slice, Kids - 1/2 slice

Ingredients:

- 3 large oranges, boiled until soft

- 4 eggs
- 1 cup almond flour
- 1 cup ground almonds
- 1/2 cup honey or agave nectar
- 1 teaspoon baking powder
- 1/2 teaspoon almond extract
- Powdered sugar for dusting (optional)

Instructions:

1. Preheat your oven to 350°F (175°C). Grease a round cake pan.
2. Cut the boiled oranges into chunks and remove any seeds.
3. In a food processor, blend the oranges until they form a smooth puree.
4. In a large mixing bowl, beat the eggs and honey or agave nectar until well combined.
5. Add the almond flour, ground almonds, baking powder, and almond extract to the egg mixture, mixing until smooth.
6. Fold in the orange puree and mix until fully incorporated.
7. Pour the batter into the greased cake pan.

8. Bake the orange and almond cake for 45-50 minutes or until a toothpick inserted into the center comes out clean.

9. Let the cake cool in the pan for 10 minutes before transferring it to a wire rack to cool completely.

10. Dust the cooled cake with powdered sugar before serving, if desired.

Exploring the Spice of Indian Sweets

Indian desserts, known as "mithai," are a celebration of aromatic spices and unique flavors, often centered around milk, nuts, and dried fruits.

Coconut Ladoo:

Serving Portions: Adults - 2 ladoos, Kids - 1 ladoo

<u>Ingredients:</u>

- 2 cups unsweetened desiccated coconut
- 1/2 cup condensed milk (low-sugar option)
- 1/2 teaspoon ground cardamom
- 1/4 cup chopped pistachios or almonds for garnish

<u>**Instructions:**</u>

1. In a non-stick pan, dry roast the desiccated coconut over low heat until it turns lightly golden and aromatic.

2. Add the condensed milk and ground cardamom to the roasted coconut, stirring continuously until the mixture thickens and starts to leave the sides of the pan.

3. Remove the pan from the heat and let the mixture cool slightly.

4. Once the mixture is cool enough to handle, take small portions and roll them into round ladoos.

5. Garnish each coconut ladoo with chopped pistachios or almonds.

6. Serve the coconut ladoo at room temperature or chilled.

Chia Kheer (Indian Rice Pudding with a Twist):

Serving Portions: Adults - 1/2 cup, Kids - 1/4 cup

<u>**Ingredients:**</u>

- 1/4 cup chia seeds

- 2 cups unsweetened almond milk
- 1/4 cup honey or agave nectar
- 1/4 teaspoon ground cardamom
- 1/4 cup chopped mixed nuts (almonds, pistachios, cashews)
- Saffron strands for garnish (optional)

Instructions:

1. In a bowl, mix the chia seeds, almond milk, honey or agave nectar, and ground cardamom until well combined.
2. Cover the bowl and refrigerate the mixture for at least 4 hours or preferably overnight, allowing the chia seeds to plump up.
3. Before serving, give the chia kheer a good stir to break up any clumps.
4. Divide the kheer into individual serving cups or bowls.
5. Garnish each portion with chopped mixed nuts and a few saffron strands for an authentic touch.

Energizing Snacks: Sustaining Your Day with Goodness

When managing diabetes, it's essential to choose snacks that provide sustained energy without causing significant spikes in blood sugar levels. In this chapter, we'll explore a variety of energizing snacks designed to keep you and your kids fueled throughout the day. These snacks are not only delicious but also packed with nutrients, making them the perfect choice for maintaining stable blood sugar levels and supporting overall health.

The Importance of Energizing Snacks

Energizing snacks play a crucial role in providing your body with the necessary nutrients and sustained energy to get you through busy days.

Balancing Blood Sugar Levels:

Well-balanced snacks that combine carbohydrates, protein, and healthy fats help regulate blood sugar levels, preventing drastic fluctuations.

Combating Midday Slumps:

Energizing snacks prevent energy crashes and fatigue, ensuring you stay focused and alert throughout the day.

Wholesome Fruit and Nut Combos

Fruits and nuts are a perfect pairing for providing a quick and energizing snack that satisfies both your sweet and savory cravings.

Apple Slices with Almond Butter:

Serving Portions: Adults - 1 medium apple with 2 tablespoons of almond butter, Kids - 1/2 medium apple with 1 tablespoon of almond butter

Instructions:

1. Wash and core the apple, then slice it into thin wedges.
2. Serve the apple slices with a side of almond butter for dipping or spreading.

Banana with Peanut Butter and Chia Seeds

Serving Portions: Adults - 1 medium banana with 2 tablespoons of peanut butter and 1 teaspoon of chia seeds, Kids - 1/2 medium banana with 1 tablespoon of peanut butter and 1/2 teaspoon of chia seeds

Instructions:

1. Peel the banana and cut it in half lengthwise.
2. Spread peanut butter on the cut sides of the banana.
3. Sprinkle chia seeds over the peanut butter.

Protein-Packed Snack Ideas

Protein is essential for maintaining energy and providing a sense of fullness, making these snacks perfect for a satisfying midday boost.

Hard-Boiled Eggs with Baby Carrots

Serving Portions: Adults - 2 hard-boiled eggs with a handful of baby carrots, Kids - 1 hard-boiled egg with a small handful of baby carrots

<u>**Instructions:**</u>

1. Hard-boil the eggs and let them cool before peeling.
2. Serve the hard-boiled eggs with a side of baby carrots for crunch and added nutrients.

Greek Yogurt with Berries and Nuts

Serving Portions: Adults - 1 cup of Greek yogurt with 1/2 cup of mixed berries and 2 tablespoons of chopped nuts, Kids - 1/2 cup of Greek yogurt with 1/4 cup of mixed berries and 1 tablespoon of chopped nuts

<u>**Instructions:**</u>

In a bowl, mix Greek yogurt with mixed berries and top with chopped nuts for added texture and flavor.

Wholesome Snacks on the Go

When you're on the move, these portable and energizing snacks will keep you fueled and focused, no matter where you are.

Trail Mix:

Serving Portions: Adults - 1/2 cup, Kids - 1/4 cup

Ingredients:

- 1/4 cup almonds
- 1/4 cup walnuts or cashews
- 1/4 cup pumpkin seeds
- 1/4 cup unsweetened dried cranberries or raisins
- 1/4 cup dark chocolate chips (look for low-sugar options)

Instructions:

1. Mix all the ingredients together and divide the trail mix into individual snack bags or containers.
2. Energy Bars (Homemade):

Serving Portions: Adults - 1 bar, Kids - 1/2 bar

Ingredients:

- 1 cup rolled oats
- 1/2 cup nut butter (almond, peanut, or cashew)

- 1/3 cup honey or agave nectar
- 1/4 cup unsweetened shredded coconut
- 1/4 cup chopped nuts (walnuts, almonds, etc.)
- 1/4 cup dark chocolate chips
- 1 teaspoon vanilla extract

Instructions:

1. In a large bowl, mix together nut butter, honey or agave nectar, and vanilla extract until well combined.
2. Add rolled oats, shredded coconut, chopped nuts, and dark chocolate chips to the bowl, and stir until everything is evenly coated.
3. Press the mixture into a lined baking dish and refrigerate for at least 2 hours to set.
4. Once set, cut the mixture into bars of your desired size.

Quick and Tasty Snack Recipes

When you need an energizing snack in a hurry, these quick and tasty recipes will come to your rescue.

Avocado and Tomato Toast:

Serving Portions: Adults - 1 slice of whole-grain toast with 1/2 avocado and sliced tomatoes, Kids - 1/2 slice of whole-grain toast with 1/4 avocado and sliced tomatoes

Instructions:

1. Toast the whole-grain bread until lightly crispy.
2. Mash the avocado and spread it on the toast.
3. Top with sliced tomatoes for a refreshing finish.

Veggie Hummus Wrap

Serving Portions: Adults - 1 whole-wheat tortilla with hummus and assorted veggies, Kids - 1/2 whole-wheat tortilla with hummus and assorted veggies

Ingredients:

- 1 whole-wheat tortilla
- 2 tablespoons hummus

- Assorted veggies (sliced cucumber, bell pepper, carrot, lettuce, etc.)

<u>Instructions:</u>

1. Spread hummus on the whole-wheat tortilla.
2. Place the assorted veggies in the center of the tortilla.
3. Roll the tortilla into a wrap, and slice it into smaller portions if desired.

Celebratory Delights: Festive Treats for Special Occasions

Special occasions call for special treats, and having diabetes doesn't mean you have to miss out on the joy of celebrating with delicious desserts. In this chapter, we'll explore a collection of diabetic-friendly recipes for festive occasions. From birthdays to holidays, these delightful treats will bring a sense of celebration to your gatherings while keeping your blood sugar levels in check. Share these recipes with your loved ones, and let the festivities be filled with deliciousness and delight for both adults and kids alike.

Balancing Indulgence and Moderation

Enjoying special treats on celebratory occasions is a part of life, and it's essential to find the right balance to savor the moment without overindulging.

Mindful Eating on Special Occasions:

By practicing mindful eating, you can fully appreciate the flavors and joy of festive treats without going overboard.

Portion Control

Controlling portion sizes allows you to enjoy your favorite desserts without causing drastic spikes in blood sugar levels.

Birthday Bash: Cake and Cupcake Delights

Birthdays are a time for celebration, and what's a birthday without a delicious cake or cupcakes to mark the occasion?

Diabetic-Friendly Chocolate Cake:

Serving Portions: Adults - 1 slice, Kids - 1/2 slice

Ingredients:

- 1 1/2 cups almond flour
- 1/2 cup unsweetened cocoa powder
- 1 teaspoon baking powder
- 1/2 teaspoon baking soda

- 1/4 teaspoon salt
- 1/2 cup unsweetened applesauce
- 1/3 cup honey or agave nectar
- 3 large eggs
- 1 teaspoon pure vanilla extract
- 1/2 cup unsweetened almond milk

Instructions:

1. Preheat your oven to 350°F (175°C). Grease a round cake pan.
2. In a large mixing bowl, whisk together the almond flour, cocoa powder, baking powder, baking soda, and salt.
3. In a separate bowl, mix the applesauce, honey or agave nectar, eggs, and vanilla extract until well combined.
4. Gradually add the wet ingredients to the dry ingredients, stirring well.
5. Slowly pour in the almond milk and mix until the batter is smooth and well combined.
6. Pour the batter into the greased cake pan.

7. Bake the chocolate cake for 30-35 minutes or until a toothpick inserted into the center comes out clean.

8. Allow the cake to cool in the pan for 10 minutes before transferring it to a wire rack to cool completely.

Mini Banana Cupcakes with Cream Cheese Frosting:

Serving Portions: Adults - 2 mini cupcakes, Kids - 1 mini cupcake

<u>Ingredients:</u>

- For the cupcakes:
- 1 cup almond flour
- 1/4 cup coconut flour
- 1 teaspoon baking powder
- 1/2 teaspoon baking soda
- 1/4 teaspoon salt
- 1/4 cup unsalted butter, softened
- 1/3 cup honey or agave nectar
- 2 large eggs
- 1 teaspoon pure vanilla extract

- 1/2 cup mashed ripe bananas (about 2 small bananas)
- 1/4 cup unsweetened almond milk

<u>For the cream cheese frosting:</u>

- 1/2 cup cream cheese, softened
- 2 tablespoons honey or agave nectar
- 1/2 teaspoon pure vanilla extract

<u>Instructions:</u>

For the cupcakes:

1. Preheat your oven to 350°F (175°C). Line a mini muffin tin with paper liners.
2. In a bowl, whisk together the almond flour, coconut flour, baking powder, baking soda, and salt.
3. In a separate bowl, cream the softened butter with honey or agave nectar until fluffy.
4. Beat in the eggs one at a time, then add the vanilla extract and mashed bananas.
5. Gradually add the dry ingredients to the wet ingredients, alternating with the

unsweetened almond milk, and mix until the batter is smooth and well combined.

6. Fill each mini muffin cup about two-thirds full with the batter.

7. Bake the mini cupcakes for 12-15 minutes or until a toothpick inserted into the center comes out clean.

8. Let the cupcakes cool in the muffin tin for 5 minutes before transferring them to a wire rack to cool completely.

For the cream cheese frosting:

1. In a mixing bowl, beat the softened cream cheese with honey or agave nectar and vanilla extract until smooth and creamy.

2. Once the cupcakes have cooled, frost the tops of the mini cupcakes with the cream cheese frosting.

Holiday Extravaganza: Special Treats for Festive Seasons

Holidays are a time of joy and celebration, and these special treats will add a touch of magic to your festivities.

Diabetic-Friendly Pumpkin Pie

Serving Portions: Adults - 1 slice, Kids - 1/2 slice

<u>Ingredients:</u>

For the crust:

- 1 1/4 cups almond flour
- 1/4 cup coconut flour
- 1/4 cup unsalted butter, chilled and cubed
- 2 tablespoons honey or agave nectar

For the filling:

- 1 can (15 oz) pure pumpkin puree
- 1/2 cup unsweetened almond milk
- 1/4 cup honey or agave nectar
- 2 large eggs
- 1 teaspoon ground cinnamon
- 1/2 teaspoon ground ginger

- 1/4 teaspoon ground nutmeg
- 1/4 teaspoon ground cloves
- 1/4 teaspoon salt

<u>Instructions:</u>

For the crust:

1. Preheat your oven to 350°F (175°C). Grease a 9-inch pie dish.
2. In a food processor, pulse together the almond flour, coconut flour, chilled butter cubes, and honey or agave nectar until the mixture resembles coarse crumbs.
3. Press the mixture into the greased pie dish, forming an even layer on the bottom and up the sides.
4. Bake the crust for 10 minutes, then remove it from the oven and set it aside to cool.

For the filling:

1. In a large bowl, whisk together the pumpkin puree, almond milk, honey or agave nectar, eggs, ground cinnamon, ground ginger,

ground nutmeg, ground cloves, and salt until well combined.

2. Pour the pumpkin mixture into the pre-baked crust.

3. Bake the pumpkin pie for 40-45 minutes or until the center is set.

4. Allow the pie to cool completely before serving.

Festive Berry Trifle

Serving Portions: Adults - 1 cup, Kids - 1/2 cup

Ingredients:

- 2 cups mixed berries (strawberries, blueberries, raspberries)
- 1/4 cup honey or agave nectar
- 1 tablespoon lemon juice
- 1 cup plain Greek yogurt
- 1/2 cup heavy cream (whipped)

Instructions:

1. In a bowl, mix the mixed berries with honey or agave nectar and lemon juice.

2. In a separate bowl, fold the whipped heavy cream into the plain Greek yogurt to create a creamy mixture.

3. In individual dessert glasses or a trifle dish, layer the mixed berries and the creamy yogurt mixture.

4. Repeat the layers until you reach the top of the glass or dish.

5. Garnish the top with a few fresh berries.

6. Refrigerate the berry trifle for at least 30 minutes before serving.

Conclusion

In the world of diabetes management, enjoying delicious snacks and desserts can often feel like a distant dream. However, with the array of diabetic-friendly snack and dessert recipes presented in this book, that dream becomes a delightful reality for both kids and adults. These recipes prove that diabetes doesn't mean sacrificing the joy of indulging in sweet treats or wholesome snacks.

Throughout this book, we embarked on a culinary journey, exploring the art of crafting balanced and delectable snacks that not only satisfy our taste buds but also support our health goals. We learned the importance of understanding diabetes and nutrition, navigating dietary requirements, and making smart snack choices to maintain stable blood sugar levels. The journey continued with chapters dedicated to delightful desserts that do not compromise on taste while promoting well-being.

With each chapter, we embraced the versatility of ingredients, the creativity in preparation, and the joy in savoring each bite. We celebrated the richness of Asian desserts, the lightness of Mediterranean delights, the aromatic spices of Indian sweets, and the global flavors that expanded our culinary horizons.

We also uncovered the wonders of nuts, fruits, and chocolates, redefining classic desserts without guilt. We discovered the joys of frozen pleasures in diabetic-friendly ice creams and indulged in quick and easy, no-bake delicacies perfect for busy days.

From energizing snacks to kid-friendly bites, from comfortingly classic treats to celebratory delights, these recipes bring a sense of satisfaction, mindfulness, and nourishment to every moment.

We relished the wholesomeness of baked goods and the creativity of fruity indulgences, each recipe designed to cater to both adults and kids, fostering a spirit of togetherness in families managing diabetes.

With portion sizes clearly outlined for adults and kids alike, these recipes ensure that each bite is a thoughtful choice, offering the perfect balance of nutrients and flavors. They empower us to embrace a holistic approach to diabetes management, where good food becomes the foundation of a healthy and fulfilling lifestyle.

As we close this culinary journey, let us remember that diabetes management need not be synonymous with deprivation. Rather, it is an opportunity to savor life's delights while making mindful and delicious choices. With these recipes in hand, we can celebrate our favorite occasions, share joy with loved ones, and embark on a journey where sweet indulgence and well-being go hand in hand.

So, let's take these diabetic-friendly snack and dessert recipes and embark on our delicious adventure—one bite at a time. Embrace the pleasure of taste, the richness of ingredients, and the joy of shared moments. Let this book serve as your companion on the path to healthier, happier, and tastier celebrations for all—kids and adults alike. Here's to the delight of diabetic-friendly treats, making every day a delicious celebration of life.

www.ingramcontent.com/pod-product-compliance
Lightning Source LLC
Chambersburg PA
CBHW060107260726

48658CB00004B/1438